PROSTATE CANCER

EXPLORING ALL FORMS OF TREATMENTS

FOR PROSTATE CANCER

DR. J. WALLER

Contents

INTRODUCTION

One type of cancer that arises in the prostate is prostate cancer. The prostate is a tiny gland that resembles a walnut that is situated in front of the rectum and beneath the bladder in males. During ejaculation, the prostate gland secretes a fluid that feeds and moves sperm.

One of the most prevalent diseases in males is prostate cancer, yet many of these instances grow slowly and may not pose a serious threat. On the other hand, malignant prostate cancers have the potential to spread to other body areas.

Age (risk rises with age), family history, race (African American males are more likely to get prostate cancer), and some genetic variables are risk factors for prostate cancer. Although the precise etiology of prostate cancer is unknown, hormonal fluctuations, prostatic inflammation, and genetics may all play a role in its development.

Prostate-specific antigen (PSA) blood tests and digital rectal exams (DREs) are common screening procedures used to identify early-stage prostate cancer, which may not exhibit any symptoms at all. Prostate cancer in its advanced stages can cause symptoms such as blood in the urine, erectile dysfunction, trouble urinating, and bone discomfort.

Prostate cancer treatment options are contingent upon a number of criteria, such as the patient's general health, the tumor's aggressiveness, and the cancer's stage. Treatment options include hormone therapy, radiation therapy, chemotherapy, active surveillance, surgery, and/or a combination of these.

The early detection and successful treatment of prostate cancer depend heavily on routine tests and knowledge of risk factors. To effectively navigate the hurdles of prostate cancer diagnosis and treatment, as with any cancer, a multidisciplinary approach incorporating medical professionals, emotional support, and well-informed decision-making is essential.

CHAPTER ONE

What Prostate Cancer Is Definition

A particular kind of cancer called prostate cancer arises in the prostate, a little gland found in the male reproductive system. The prostate is located in front of the rectum and directly beneath the bladder. The production of seminal fluid, a nutrient-rich fluid that feeds and moves sperm during ejaculation, is its main job.

Tumors are formed when the prostate gland's cells grow abnormally and uncontrollably. This is known as prostate cancer. Although it is one of the most prevalent malignancies in males, most instances grow slowly and may not pose a serious threat to health. On the other hand, malignant prostate cancers have the potential to spread to other body areas.

Although the precise etiology of prostate cancer is unknown, there are some risk factors that are linked to the disease's development. These include race (African American men having a higher risk), family history, age (with the risk increasing as men age), and genetic variables.

Prostate-specific antigen (PSA) blood tests and digital rectal exams (DREs) are common screening procedures used to identify early-stage prostate cancer, which may not exhibit any symptoms at all. Advanced stages may show symptoms such as blood in the urine, erectile dysfunction, trouble urinating, or bone discomfort.

Prostate cancer treatment options are contingent upon various circumstances, including the patient's overall health, the tumor's aggressiveness, and the cancer's stage. Treatment options could involve radiation therapy, hormone therapy, chemotherapy, active surveillance, surgery, or a mix of these.

The early detection and successful treatment of prostate cancer depend heavily on routine tests and knowledge of risk factors. In order to effectively manage the issues associated with prostate cancer, a complete and tailored approach incorporating healthcare specialists, emotional support, and informed decision-making is important.

A little gland that resembles a walnut, the prostate is a component of the male reproductive system. It surrounds the urethra, the tube that takes semen from the reproductive system out through the penis and urine from the bladder, and is situated directly below the bladder, in front of the rectum. The prostate is engaged in many body processes and is essential to the reproductive process.

Inside the Prostate: Anatomy

The prostate gland is separated into zones and has multiple lobes:

Prostate cancer most frequently develops in the peripheral zone, which is the outermost portion of the prostate.

Transition Zone: This area, which encircles the urethra, is in charge of the prostate's expansion, which frequently happens as people age and results in benign prostatic hyperplasia (BPH).

The central zone, which encircles the ejaculatory ducts, is less frequently linked to prostate cancer.

The prostate's function:

The prostate gland plays a number of crucial roles in the male reproductive system, including:

Generation of Seminal Fluid: The prostate's main job is to generate a large amount of the seminal fluid that combines with sperm during ejaculation. Sperm benefit from this fluid's protection and nourishment, which helps them endure in the female reproductive system.

Muscular Contractions: During ejaculation, the muscles of the prostate gland assist in pushing semen into the urethra. The body expels semen with the help of this procedure.

Prostate-specific antigen (PSA) is one of the enzymes produced by the prostate that liquefies semen following ejaculation. In diagnostic tests, PSA is also utilized as a marker for prostate health.

Impact on Urination: The prostate's surrounding the urethra makes it a potential source of influence on urination. Prostate enlargement

(BPH) can compress the urethra, making it difficult to urinate.

The prostate's main function is reproduction, although it can also develop benign prostatic hyperplasia and prostate cancer, among other diseases. Prostate health maintenance and prompt resolution of any potential concerns require routine check-ups, screenings, and awareness of possible signs.

Hazard Contributors

Prostate cancer may arise as a result of multiple risk factors. Individuals can assess their risk and take necessary action by having a better understanding of these elements. It's crucial to remember that the presence of one or more risk factors does not ensure the development of prostate cancer; in fact, people without obvious risk factors may nonetheless receive a diagnosis of the illness. The following are some typical prostate cancer risk factors:

Age: As people age, their chance of prostate cancer rises. Prostate cancer is uncommon in males under 40, but beyond age 50, the risk increases dramatically. Men over 65 are diagnosed with the majority of instances.

Family History: Those who had a father or brother who was a first-degree relative who also had prostate cancer are more likely to have the disease. If the condition was discovered at an earlier age or if more relatives are afflicted, the risk is increased.

Race/Ethnicity: Compared to men of other races, African American men are more likely to develop prostate cancer. Asian American and Hispanic/Latino guys are less likely to have it. It's unclear why there are racial differences in this way.

Genetic Factors: A higher risk of prostate cancer may result from inherited genetic alterations. An increased risk of prostate cancer has been connected to mutations in specific genes, such as BRCA1 and BRCA2, which are linked to ovarian and breast malignancies.

Geographic Location: Prostate cancer incidence varies by region, with greater rates found in Australia, Europe, and North America. In Africa and Asia, it is less widespread.

Dietary Factors: Studies have indicated that a diet heavy in processed and red meats and low in fruits and vegetables may raise the risk of prostate cancer, however the exact relationship between the two is unclear. A diet high in fruits and vegetables provides antioxidants, which may offer some protection.

Obesity: Some data point to a possible link between obesity and a higher risk of aggressive types of prostate cancer.

Occupational Exposures: A number of occupational exposures have been proposed as possible risk factors for prostate cancer, including exposure to cadmium or agent orange.

Prostate Inflammation: Prostatitis, or persistent inflammation of the prostate, has been linked to a higher risk of prostate cancer.

It's critical that people understand their risk factors and talk to medical professionals about them. Prostate cancer can be identified at an early, more treatable stage with regular screenings and early detection with tests like the digital rectal exam (DRE) and the prostate-specific antigen (PSA) blood test.

Symptoms and Indications

Prostate cancer frequently exhibits no signs in its early stages. However, some people may develop symptoms and signs as the malignancy worsens. It is noteworthy that there are other noncancerous illnesses that might potentially be linked to same symptoms. Seeking further assessment from a healthcare expert is advised if any of these symptoms worsen or continue. Prostate cancer symptoms and indicators frequently include:

Changes in Urine:

difficulty starting or halting the flow of pee.

weak or irregular flow of pee.

frequent urine, particularly during the evening (nocturia).

a strong need to urinate.

Blood in Semen or Urine:

hemoturia, or the presence of blood in the urine, or semen.

Ineffective Penis:

inability to obtain or sustain an erection.

Pelvic Pain:

ache or discomfort in the upper thighs, lower back, or pelvis.

Bone Aches:

Prostate cancer that has progressed to an advanced stage may cause bone discomfort, particularly in the hips, spine, and pelvis.

Fatigue with Loss of Weight:

unaccounted-for weight loss.

ongoing exhaustion.

It's crucial to stress that benign diseases like prostatitis or benign prostatic hyperplasia (BPH) can also induce these symptoms; they are not exclusive to prostate cancer. Furthermore, it is possible for prostate cancer in its early stages to not exhibit any symptoms, which emphasizes the significance of routine testing for early identification.

A digital rectal examination (DRE) and a prostate-specific antigen (PSA) blood test are frequently used in conjunction for routine screenings for prostate cancer. A prostate biopsy or other additional diagnostic procedures may be necessary to confirm or rule out the existence of cancer if elevated PSA levels or other abnormalities found during a DRE are found.

Prostate cancer screening schedules and frequency should be discussed with healthcare practitioners for individuals who have risk factors, such as age, family history, or genetic susceptibility. For those with prostate cancer, early identification and timely medical intervention can lead to more successful therapy and improved prognoses.

Identifying and Preventing

Prostate cancer must be screened for and detected early in order to be treated more effectively. Choosing to get screened for prostate cancer requires taking into account personal preferences, risk factors, and conversations with medical professionals. The following are typical techniques for prostate cancer screening:

Blood Test for Prostate-Specific Antigen (PSA):

The prostate gland secretes the protein known as PSA. The amount of PSA in the blood is determined by a PSA blood test.

Prostate cancer is one of the illnesses that elevated PSA values can signify. On the other hand, benign diseases like prostatitis or benign prostatic hyperplasia (BPH) can also cause increased PSA values.

Because of its imperfections, the PSA test may produce false positives or false negatives. In addition, PSA levels can be influenced by age, race, and medication.

Rectal Exam Digital (DRE):

A doctor does a DRE by putting a gloved, lubricated finger inside the rectum to feel for lumps or hard spots in the prostate.

The size, shape, and texture of the prostate can be accurately determined by DRE, even though it is less sensitive than the PSA test.

For a more thorough evaluation, the PSA test and DRE are frequently administered together.

mpMRI stands for multiparametric magnetic resonance imaging.

A variety of magnetic resonance imaging (MRI) sequences are combined in mpMRI to produce detailed images of the prostate.

It is becoming more and more common to evaluate the prostate and direct focused biopsies, particularly when there are increased PSA values or questionable results.

Prostate Biopsy:

Prostate biopsies could be advised if screening tests for prostate cancer, such PSA and DRE, indicate a possible risk.

Little tissue samples from the prostate gland are removed during a biopsy, and they are analyzed under a microscope to identify any cancer and confirm its presence.

CHAPTER TWO

Genetic Examination:

Genetic testing may be considered in certain circumstances, particularly for those with a family history of prostate cancer or certain genetic risk factors.

A comprehensive discussion with healthcare experts over the decision to have a prostate cancer screening should take into account various considerations, including age, general health, family history, and personal preferences. There are some hazards associated with screening, and false positive results may cause needless worry and actions. On the other hand, erroneous negative results could postpone cancer diagnosis.

There may be differences in screening protocols, so people should talk to their healthcare professionals about the advantages and drawbacks of screening in order to make an informed decision that fits their particular situation. For continued prostate health, regular follow-up and discussion with medical professionals are crucial.

Identification

A number of procedures and medical exams are involved in the diagnosis of prostate cancer in order to establish the disease's existence, identify its features, and inform treatment choices. An outline of the prostate cancer diagnosis procedure is provided below:

Exams for screening:

Digital rectal examinations (DREs) and blood testing for the prostate-specific antigen (PSA) are two common screening procedures that lead the diagnosis process.

Extra inquiries may be necessary in response to aberrant findings or elevated PSA levels during a DRE.

mpMRI stands for multiparametric magnetic resonance imaging.

mpMRI is a sophisticated imaging method that yields fine-grained prostate pictures.

Targeted biopsies can be guided by mpMRI, which can also assist in identifying prostate cancerous regions.

Prostate Biopsy:

A prostate biopsy could be suggested if imaging or screening tests point to a possible risk of prostate cancer.

Using a fine needle, little tissue samples are extracted from the prostate during a biopsy. After that, the samples are inspected under a microscope to check for the presence of cancer and evaluate its features, including the Gleason score, which indicates how aggressive the cancer is.

Gleason Rating:

A grading system called the Gleason score is used to determine how aggressive prostate cancer is. The emergence of cancer cells in the biopsy samples serves as the basis for this.

Higher scores indicate more aggressive cancer. The Gleason score goes from 6 to 10.

Setting:

Prostate cancer is staged to ascertain the extent of its spread after a diagnosis is made. Treatment choices are guided in part by staging.

Imaging studies like bone scans, CT scans, or MRIs may be used in staging to determine whether the cancer has progressed beyond the prostate.

Genetic Examination:

Under certain circumstances, genetic testing might be taken into consideration, particularly if there is a family history of prostate cancer or particular genetic risk factors.

Certain genetic mutations linked to an increased risk of prostate cancer can be found by genetic testing.

Speaking with Experts:

Specialists such as urologists and oncologists work together to discuss the diagnosis and create a thorough treatment plan.

Healthcare providers from a variety of specializations work together to diagnose prostate cancer. The right course of treatment—which may involve active monitoring, surgery, radiation therapy, hormone therapy, or a combination of these—is determined in part by the data obtained from screening, imaging, biopsy, and staging.

Prostate cancer patients are advised to ask questions, participate actively in treatment plan decisions, and have honest and knowledgeable conversations with their medical team. When it comes to improving prostatic cancer patient outcomes, early identification and precise diagnosis are essential.

Prostate Cancer Types

Numerous forms and subtypes of prostate cancer exist, each with distinct characteristics, making it a varied disease. The two primary forms of prostate cancer are neuroendocrine tumors and adenocarcinomas. Most occurrences of prostate cancer are caused by the most prevalent kind, adenocarcinoma. Although they are less frequent, neuroendocrine tumors can be more aggressive. Let's examine these kinds in more detail:

Adenocarcinoma:

Description: Adenocarcinoma accounts for more than 90% of instances of prostate cancer, making it the most common kind. It starts in the prostate's glandular cells.

Gleason Score: Based on the appearance of cancer cells in biopsy samples, adenocarcinomas are given a Gleason score that denotes the aggressiveness of the malignancy.

Tumors Neuroendocrine:

Prostate neuroendocrine tumors are less prevalent but more likely to be aggressive. They could appear as an adenocarcinoma's advancement.

Aggressiveness: Prostate cancer that is neuroendocrine is frequently linked to a worse prognosis and may not react as well to conventional prostate cancer treatments.

Markers: Unlike adenocarcinomas, these tumors may not express the prostate-specific antigen (PSA) as strongly, which makes it difficult to identify them using conventional screening techniques.

Tiny Cell Cancer:

Prostate small cell carcinoma is an uncommon and aggressive form. It is classified as a type of prostate cancer that is neuroendocrine.

Aggression: Small cell carcinomas have a propensity to grow quickly and may be more likely to spread to other body areas.

Adenocarcinoma Ductal:

A kind of adenocarcinoma that develops in the prostate's ducts is called ductal adenocarcinoma.

Look: When viewed under a microscope, ductal adenocarcinomas can be distinguished from other types of adenocarcinomas by certain characteristics.

Carcinoma Sarcomatoid:

Sarcomatoid carcinoma is an uncommon and very aggressive form of prostate cancer that combines features of a sarcoma and a carcinoma.

Sarcoma-like spindle-shaped cells can be observed under a microscope in sarcomatoid carcinomas.

It's crucial to remember that prostate cancer is a heterogeneous disease, which means that different people may experience the illness in different ways. Treatment decisions are guided by the Gleason score, which evaluates the appearance of cancer cells in biopsy samples and helps determine the aggressiveness of the malignancy.

Comprehending the distinct kind and attributes of prostate cancer is imperative in formulating a customized therapy regimen that caters to the individual circumstances of the patient. Depending on the kind and stage of prostate cancer, treatment options may include surgery, radiation therapy, hormone therapy, chemotherapy, or a combination of these.

Options for Treatment

The stage and grade of the cancer, the patient's general health, and personal preferences all play a role in the treatment plan selection for prostate cancer. Prostate cancer treatment choices could involve:

Monitoring in Action:

Active surveillance entails regular check-ups, PSA tests, and sporadic biopsies to closely monitor the malignancy.

Indications: Since early-stage or low-risk prostate cancer grows slowly and may not need immediate treatment, this strategy is frequently taken into consideration.

Prostatectomy surgery:

The surgical excision of the prostate gland is known as a prostatectomy. Radiation prostatectomy, laparoscopic prostatectomy, and robotic-assisted prostatectomy are among the several forms of prostatectomies.

Indications: In cases of localized prostate cancer, especially when the cancer is contained to the prostate and has not spread, a prostatectomy is frequently advised.

Radiation Treatment:

High-energy radiation is used in radiation therapy to specifically target and destroy cancer cells. Brachytherapy (internal radiation) and external beam radiation are two forms of radiation therapy for prostate cancer.

Indications: Radiation therapy can be administered as an adjuvant therapy following surgery or as the main treatment for localized prostate cancer.

Androgen Deprivation Therapy (Hormone Therapy):

The goal of hormone therapy is to reduce or stop the synthesis of androgens, or male hormones, which are known to promote the growth of prostate cancer cells. Examples of these hormones include testosterone.

Indications: For advanced or metastatic prostate cancer, hormone therapy may be combined with other forms of treatment. To increase the efficacy of radiation therapy, it can also be used beforehand.

Chemotherapy:

Drugs are used in chemotherapy to either kill or slow the growth of cancer cells. When prostate cancer has progressed and other treatments may not be effective, it is usually employed.

Indications: In cases of metastatic prostate cancer or in cases when alternative therapies have failed, chemotherapy may be advised.

Immunotherapy:

Immunotherapy activates the immune system to identify and combat cancerous cells. It is a more recent method of treating advanced prostate cancer.

Indications: Patients with metastatic prostate cancer may be candidates for immunotherapy.

CHAPTER THREE

Specialized Treatments:

Medications known as "targeted therapies" aim to target cancer cells or the environment around them. They could be applied in addition to other therapies.

Indications: If an advanced prostate cancer has developed resistance to hormonal therapy, targeted therapies may be a viable option.

Therapies Aimed at the Bone:

To help control bone pain and problems, certain drugs are particularly made to target bone metastases linked to advanced prostate cancer.

Indications: For metastatic prostate cancer, bone-targeted medicines may be used with other forms of treatment.

Patients are advised to explore their options with their healthcare team, which includes urologists, radiation oncologists, medical oncologists, and other specialists, as treatment decisions are extremely customized. The process of selecting decisions may entail taking the patient's preferences and general health into account in addition to the possible advantages, dangers, and side effects of each treatment.

Dietary assistance

A supplementary role for nutritional support can be played in the overall care and wellbeing of patients with prostate cancer. Even while everyone should eat a healthy, balanced diet, there are several dietary practices that can support prostate health and even improve the results of medical therapies. The following dietary guidelines are suggested for those who have prostate cancer:

Consume a Healthy Diet:

Have a diet rich in whole grains, lean meats, healthy fats, and a variety of fruits and vegetables. Essential elements for general health can be obtained via a varied diet.

Rich in Antioxidants Foods:

Incorporate antioxidant-rich foods including leafy green vegetables, almonds, citrus fruits, and berries. Antioxidants may aid in preventing cell damage.

The Fatty Acids Omega-3:

Include foods high in omega-3 fatty acids, like walnuts, flaxseeds, chia seeds, and fatty fish (salmon, mackerel, and sardines). Omega-3s have the ability to reduce inflammation.

Cut Back on Processed and Red Meats:

Red and processed meats should be consumed in moderation since they have been linked to a higher risk of prostate cancer. Select sources of lean protein, such as fish, chicken, beans, and lentils.

Cruciferous Squash:

Add veggies that belong to the cruciferous family, like Brussels sprouts, broccoli, cauliflower, and cabbage. Certain chemicals found in these veggies may have anti-cancer properties.

Lycopene and tomatoes:

One of the strongest antioxidants, lycopene, may be found in tomatoes. Tomato cooking can improve lycopene absorption. Think about including goods made from cooked tomatoes in your diet.

And isoflavones in soy:

Isoflavones, which are found in soy products like tofu and edamame, may have protective benefits. Nevertheless, research on soy's potential connection to prostate cancer is still underway, and individual results may differ.

Green Tea:

Polyphenols found in green tea, such as catechins, have anti-oxidant qualities. Prostate health may benefit, according to certain research.

Sustain a Healthy Weight:

It's critical to reach and maintain a healthy weight because obesity has been associated with a higher chance of developing aggressive prostate cancer.

Drinking plenty of water

Make sure you are properly hydrated by consuming enough water. Maintaining adequate hydration is critical to general health.

Speak with a Certified Dietitian:

If you would like individualized food suggestions based on your specific needs, treatment plan, and probable side effects, speak with a certified dietician with expertise in cancer.

Prostate cancer patients should always consult their medical team before making any major dietary or supplemental changes. The precise kind and stage of prostate cancer, as well as individual medical conditions and treatment regimens, may all influence dietary decisions. Prostate cancer patients can benefit from a team approach that incorporates medical and dietary advice to improve their overall health.

Survival and Aftercare

Prostate cancer survivorship entails continued surveillance, post-treatment care, and managing the psychological and physical aspects of life. The following are important facets of follow-up care and survivorship for people who have finished treatment for prostate cancer:

Recheck Appointments:

Keep your follow-up appointments with your medical team on a regular basis. Check-ups, blood testing (including PSA tests), and conversations regarding any worries or symptoms may be part of these appointments.

Tracking PSA Levels:

After therapy, PSA levels are frequently checked for any indications of recurrence. Your healthcare professional will decide how often you need to get PSA tests.

Taking Care of Side Effects of Treatment:

Talk about any new or persistent adverse effects with your medical provider. These might involve problems with bowel habits, sexual health, and urine function. Support or interventions that are appropriate can be given.

Sustaining an Invigorating Lifestyle:

Maintaining a healthy weight, exercising frequently, and adhering to a balanced diet should all remain top priorities in a healthy lifestyle. These elements support general well-being and may have a favorable effect on long-term health.

Support for Mental and Emotional Health:

For your mental and emotional health, get help. Survivorship can elicit a range of feelings, therefore it might be helpful to speak with counselors, medical professionals, or support groups.

Bone Well-being:

Bone health may be a factor for those undergoing androgen deprivation therapy (hormone therapy). Talk about ways to keep your bones healthy, such as taking supplements of calcium and vitamin D if necessary.

Sexual Wellness:

Talk with your healthcare team about options for managing and enhancing sexual health if your treatment has affected your ability to have sex. Medication, therapy, or other interventions might be part of this.

Dealing with the Fear of Recurrence:

A common anxiety among survivors is that of cancer coming back. Having open lines of communication with medical professionals and voicing concerns can help control anxiety and enhance general quality of life.

Plans for Long-Term Survivorship Care:

Create a survivorship care plan with your medical team that details suggested testing, follow-up care, and lifestyle advice based on your individual circumstances.

Frequent Workout:

Regular physical activity has been shown to have a number of health benefits. Exercise lowers the chance of developing various medical disorders, enhances mood, and helps preserve strength.

Education and Advocacy:

Keep abreast on developments in the diagnosis, treatment, and prevention of prostate cancer. Making decisions about your health that are well-informed can be achieved by speaking up for yourself and taking advantage of educational opportunities.

Social Assistance:

Keep in touch with your loved ones, friends, and support networks. Having social support is essential for maintaining emotional health during the surviving stage.

Prostate cancer survivorship necessitates a comprehensive strategy that takes into account not just the physical but also the psychological and emotional facets of health. A good survivorship experience is influenced by maintaining regular contact with healthcare providers, adhering to follow-up care plans, and placing an emphasis on general well-being.

Strategies for Prevention and Lifestyle

Prostate cancer risk can be decreased by leading a healthy lifestyle and putting preventive measures into place. Although it is not possible to prevent every instance of prostate cancer, adopting these lifestyle habits could potentially enhance general prostate health. The following are some preventative and lifestyle tips:

Keep Up a Nutritional Diet:

Eat a diet high in fruits, vegetables, whole grains, lean proteins, and balance. Fruits and vegetables contain antioxidants, which may offer protective benefits.

Cut Back on Processed and Red Meats:

Reduce your consumption of red and processed meats because they have been linked to a higher risk of prostate cancer. Opt for lean protein sources including poultry, fish, beans, and legumes.

Add Good Fats:

Include sources of good fats, like walnuts, flaxseeds, chia seeds, and omega-3 fatty acids, which are found in fatty fish.

Lycopene and tomatoes:

Consume lycopene, a potent antioxidant with potential prostate-protective properties, by include tomatoes and tomato-based items in your diet.

CHAPTER FOUR

Cruciferous Squash:

Eat cruciferous veggies, which may contain anti-cancer qualities. Examples of these vegetables are broccoli, cauliflower, cabbage, and Brussels sprouts.

And isoflavones in soy:

Add to your diet soy products like edamame and tofu, as they contain isoflavones that may protect the prostate.

Sustain a Healthy Weight:

Reach and stay at a healthy weight by eating a balanced diet and engaging in regular physical activity. An increased risk of aggressive prostate cancer has been associated with obesity.

Frequent Workout:

Exercise on a regular basis, focusing on strength and aerobic conditioning. Try to get in at least 150 minutes a week of moderate-to-intense activity.

Maintain Hydration:

To be properly hydrated, consume enough water. Staying well hydrated promotes general health.

Limit Your Alcohol Consumption:

Restrict alcohol intake because too much of it has been linked to a higher risk of prostate cancer.

Give Up Smoking:

Give up smoking if you do. There are multiple cancers for which smoking is a risk factor, and there are many health advantages of stopping.

Frequent examinations and screenings:

Make an appointment for routine check-ups with your healthcare provider and talk about the proper prostate cancer tests, particularly if your age, family history, or other circumstances put you at higher risk.

Control Your Stress:

Try stress-relieving exercises like yoga, mindfulness, or meditation. General health may be impacted by ongoing stress.

Reduce Your Toxin Exposure in the Environment:

Take care not to come into contact with chemicals and pesticides, among other environmental pollutants. When at all possible, minimize exposure.

Genetic Guidance:

To determine your personal risk and possible preventive steps, think about genetic counseling if you have a family history of prostate cancer or other risk factors.

It's crucial to remember that different people may react differently to lifestyle modifications, and using these tactics won't ensure that prostate cancer won't develop. On the other hand, leading a healthy lifestyle can improve general wellbeing and lower the chance of developing a number of illnesses, such as prostate cancer. Always seek the opinion of medical specialists for individualized guidance unique to your health status and risk factors.

Effects on Emotion and Psychology

People with prostate cancer may experience severe emotional and psychological effects that negatively impact different facets of their wellbeing. Prostate cancer-related emotional difficulties can include:

Anxiety & Fear:

A prostate cancer diagnosis can cause worry and anxiety due to treatment outcomes, daily life effects, and future uncertainties.

Depression

Depressive, gloomy, and depressing feelings might surface, especially while dealing with the psychological effects of a cancer diagnosis and the difficulties of therapy.

Angry and Exasperated:

Some people may become angry or frustrated when their plans for their lives are upset, when relationships are impacted, or when they face both physical and psychological difficulties while receiving therapy.

Issues with Body Image:

Prostate cancer treatments like radiation or surgery might alter one's body image and impair one's ability to have sexual relations. Emotionally, adjusting to these changes can be difficult.

Problems with Intimacy:

Relationship tension can result from changes in closeness and sexual function. Addressing issues with intimacy requires being transparent in communicating and asking for help when needed.

Effect on Interpersonal Relationships:

Relationships with partners, family, and friends may be impacted by prostate cancer. It might bring up new dynamics, and overcoming the obstacles might call for candid communication.

Sadness and Loss:

A cancer diagnosis might cause one to feel as though they have lost something important in life, such as their health or their imagined invulnerability.

Vacancy Regarding the Future:

Stress and emotional strain might result from having to live with the uncertainty of cancer and its possible recurrence. It can be difficult to deal with the unknown parts of the future.

Changes in Roles:

It may be necessary for people and their support systems to adapt to new roles, such as that of caregiver or cancer survivor.

Stress Related to Money:

Stress and worry can be exacerbated by the cost of cancer treatment, medical expenses, and possible job changes.

Social Detachment:

Some people may socially disengage because they feel ashamed or embarrassed, or because they want to shield their loved ones from hardship.

Effective Coping Techniques:

Positively, people might learn coping mechanisms, resilience, and a fresh perspective on life. Discovering purpose and meaning can be a part of the journey that follows diagnosis.

Prostate cancer has an emotional and psychological toll, and getting support from loved ones, friends, mental health experts, and medical professionals is crucial. The promotion of candid communication, the pursuit of therapy or counseling, and the inclusion of family members in the supportive care regimen can all enhance emotional health both during and after cancer treatment. In addition, stress-reduction methods, mindfulness exercises, and an emphasis on general self-care can help to foster emotional resilience.

Due to the complexity and diversity of prostate cancer, diagnosis, treatment, and survivability all need to be approached from an all-encompassing perspective. It is the second most prevalent type of cancer in males worldwide, and its effects go beyond the physical to include social, psychological, and emotional components.

Treatment outcomes are greatly enhanced by early discovery through screening, such as PSA tests and digital rectal exams. Knowing risk variables, such as age, genetic inclination, and family history, makes it easier to identify those who might benefit from routine screening.

Treatment regimens that are specific to each patient are necessary due to the wide range of prostate cancer forms, which include neuroendocrine tumors and adenocarcinomas. Treatment options are tailored to the specifics of each case and include active surveillance, surgery, radiation therapy, hormone therapy, and newer immunotherapies.

In order to support general well-being, survivorship entails continual monitoring, support, and lifestyle modifications. Healthcare professionals, support groups, and loved ones must provide attention and support for emotional and psychological issues like fear, anxiety, and changes in body image.

Prostate cancer risk can be decreased by adopting preventive measures such a nutritious diet, consistent exercise, and lifestyle changes. The field of prostate cancer care is still being shaped by developments in treatment options, early detection, and genetic counseling.

Prostate cancer knowledge and viable interventions will change as science and medicine move forward. In order to effectively treat prostate cancer, it is imperative that people are empowered with knowledge, that awareness be raised, and that patients and healthcare professionals work together.

In the end, overcoming prostate cancer requires fortitude, optimism, and the combined efforts of sufferers, medical professionals, researchers, and support systems. Prostate cancer outcomes and quality of life can be improved, and ultimately a cure can be found, with sustained research, activism, and holistic care.

THE END

www.ingramcontent.com/pod-product-compliance
Lightning Source LLC
Chambersburg PA
CBHW050851260726
48660CB00006B/2560